Pilates and Jesus

Strengthening the Body, Mind, and Spirit

Table of Contents

Chapter 1. Introduction

Welcome to our Special Report: Pilates and Jesus: Strengthening the Body, Mind, and Spirit! This delightful exploration takes you on a journey through the converging paths of physical well-being and spiritual rejuvenation. Combining the toning, core-centered approach of Pilates with the profound spiritual teachings of Jesus, this report offers a unique and enriching perspective on holistic wellness. Embrace an invigorating reading experience that's set to rejuvenate you from within, and inspire an enhanced living—strengthening not just your muscles, but also your faith and intellect. Let's embark on this harmonious communion of body, mind, and spirit together, and enrich our lives with newfound vitality. We promise, that after perusing through this report, you will feel refreshed, revitalized, and truly connected to your inner self and divine beliefs. Don't miss this opportunity—Gift yourself a whole new perspective on comprehensive wellness today!

Chapter 2. The Intersection of Pilates and Spirituality

Even though the exploration of the intersection between Pilates and spirituality might seem like a novel idea, these two disciplines have significant commonalities. The underlying principles of Pilates—centering, control, flow, breath, precision, and concentration—mirror some critical aspects of various spiritual traditions. This chapter will delve into the combined power of Pilates and spirituality and show you how this union can bring about holistic health and wellness.

2.1. A Brief Overview of Pilates

Joseph Pilates, the creator of Pilates, was keenly focused on the unity of body, mind, and spirit. Trained in gymnastics, bodybuilding, and yoga, Pilates developed his unique fitness methodology in the early 20th century. He believed the body and mind were closely connected and that training both could alleviate everyday physical and emotional problems.

Pilates is a fitness system designed to improve physical strength, flexibility, and posture, and enhance mental awareness. It focuses on the 'powerhouse'—the collective term for the abdominals, lower and upper back, hips, buttocks, and inner thighs. These are the core muscles that Pilates targets, helping individuals maintain balance and develop strength.

2.2. Jesus and Spirituality

On the other hand, Jesus's teachings outline a spiritual life centered around love, compassion, forgiveness, service, and a personal relationship with God. Spirituality, as encapsulated by Jesus, advises turning inward, understanding the self, recognizing one's weaknesses, and aspiring for growth and transformation.

2.3. The Interconnection: Pilates and Spirituality

Both Pilates and spiritual teachings advocate for an inner journey. Whereas Pilates concentrates on the inner body—enhancing the core, improving flexibility, and promoting overall fitness—spiritual discourse, like that exemplified by Jesus, spotlights development and wellness of the mind and the spirit.

Both domains emphasize mindfulness, too. Pilates practitioners develop mindfulness through conscious movements aimed at engaging specific muscles. Similarly, spirituality encourages mindfulness in thoughts, actions, and interactions.

2.4. The Role of Breath

Breath acts as another common thread that binds Pilates and spirituality. In Pilates, the importance of breath cannot be overstated—it powers the exercises, helps in engaging the core, and even aids in enhancing stability and balance. Likewise, spiritual traditions also underscore the role of breath in meditation—controlling it helps clear the mind, balance emotions, and achieve tranquility.

2.5. Building Strength and Flexibility—Physical and Spiritual

Regular Pilates practice builds not only physical strength but also mental endurance as one learns to push through challenging exercises. It is a path to physical flexibility; it also opens the mind to the idea of overcoming obstacles, fostering mental and emotional flexibility.

In the spiritual context, strength is about having the courage to face life's challenges, persist through difficulties, and uphold one's faith. Flexibility pertains to the capacity to adapt to life's twists and turns, demonstrating resilience and openness to new perspectives.

2.6. Beyond the Physical: Pilates and Mental Wellness

Pilates, though primarily known for its physical benefits, contributes significantly to mental wellness, too. The practice demands complete concentration, helping individuals keep out distracting thoughts, thereby fostering mindfulness and relaxation. It bolsters emotional health by reducing stress, calming the mind, and increasing body awareness.

With its emphasis on balance and control, Pilates also aids in enhancing body image and promoting positive self-perception. Meanwhile, spiritual teachings of Jesus advocate for unconditional self-love and acceptance, complementing the boosts to mental wellness provided by Pilates.

2.7. The Ultimate Goal: Rejuvenation and Transformation of the Whole Being

The union of Pilates and spirituality aims to rejuvenate and transform the whole person. By reinforcing each other, they try to promote a comprehensive sense of well-being across the three dimensions of human selfhood: body, mind, and spirit. The reward is a healthier, flexible, stronger, and more balanced individual, demonstrating greater resilience and adaptability in the face of life's challenges.

2.8. The Practice

How, then, does one combine Pilates and spirituality in practice? It begins with setting an intention, whether it's developing strength, achieving serene peace of mind, or cultivating emotional resilience. As your Pilates routine guides you through mindful movements, integrate spiritual practices such as prayer, meditation, or contemplation. You might meditate on a teaching of Jesus during a Pilates session, reflect upon it as you engage your core and breath, and then carry this wisdom into your interactions beyond the mat.

In the end, the intersection of Pilates and spirituality enlightens us about the profound interconnectedness of our beings—body, mind, and spirit. It underscores that caring for one, we care for all; neglecting one, we neglect all. The harmonious convergence of these disciplines persuades us to pursue a holistic approach towards wellness—an approach enhancing not just physical strength or flexibility, but also nourishing the soul, enlightening the intellect, and encouraging an uplifted spirit. The journey, undoubtedly challenging at times, promises immense growth and fulfillment—worth every bead of sweat and every moment of introspection.

Chapter 3. Origin of Pilates: Genesis and Goal

In the early 20th century, a remarkable fitness regimen emerged on the horizon of exercise—Pilates. This distinctive approach to physical well-being was conceived by one man, Joseph Hubertus Pilates. Born in 1883 in Mönchengladbach, Germany, Joseph's early life was fraught with ailments such as rickets, asthma and rheumatic fever. His frail health set him on a relentless quest for physical improvement, a pursuit that ultimately birthed the Pilates method.

3.1. Joseph Pilates: The Genesis of an Innovator

As a child, Pilates demonstrated a voracious curiosity about the human body. He studied both Eastern and Western forms of exercise to understand their underlying principle, dissect anatomy books to grasp the mechanics of musculature and movement, and disciplined himself in yoga, martial arts, gymnastics, skiing, and boxing to train his body. He began to see the body as an integrated whole—where strenuous physical activity was harmoniously accompanied by conscious thought and deliberate, flowing movement.

During World War I, Pilates was interned in Britain along with other German nationals. During this time, he served as an orderly in a hospital, dealing with patients unable to walk. He recognized the necessity of an exercise regimen that could be done even in a prone position. Combining his knowledge about exercise and the human anatomy, he began devising equipment with springs attached to hospital beds. These contraptions were the rudimentary precursors to today's high-tech Pilates equipment. They allowed bedridden patients to exercise their muscles without strain.

3.2. Pilates Method: The Goal

Joseph Pilates believed in his method's holistic healing power and the integral relationship between mind and body. He maintained that the quality of every movement mattered more than the number of times the movement was performed. This echoes the view of mindfulness in every action, a deeply spiritual approach to everyday life.

Pilates named his method 'Contrology.' He defined Contrology as "the comprehensive integration of body, mind, and spirit." This ideology seems to mirror the teachings of Jesus, who advocated an integrated life—physically, mentally, and spiritually—to experience the abundant life that he promised.

At the core of Pilates lies a set of principles, often referred to as six Pilates principles - concentration, control, center, flow, precision and breathing.

Concentration encourages the practitioner to stay mindful and conscious of each movement they perform. This mental engagement is vital to gain maximum benefits from the exercises.

Control, or, as Pilates referred to it, 'Contrology', refers to maintaining a mindful command of your muscles to perform movements with maximum benefit and minimal strain.

Center denotes the focal point of the Pilates workout. Every movement in a Pilates workout initiates from the center (the core muscles) and flows outward to the extremities.

Flow stands for fluidity and grace with which the exercises are performed. Pilates emphasized that his exercises should be carried out with the elegance and smoothness of a ballet dancer.

Precision is the key to achieving the desired results. Each exercise is performed with meticulous attention to detail.

Breathing aims to cleanse the body and maintain a rhythmic coordination with physical movements. Pilates recommended deep, controlled breathing to increase oxygen intake.

3.3. Pilates: Harmonizing Exercise with Holistic Wellness

The philosophical underpinnings of Pilates don't merely point to physical exercise, but interestingly align with the spiritual teachings of Jesus Christ. The focus on a calm, concentrated mind resonates with Christ's teachings about peace, while the precise, controlled movements remind one of Jesus's deliberateness in his ministry. The integration of physical effort with conscious awareness is akin to how Jesus led a life of purpose and thoughtfulness.

Just as Christ spread His teachings to foster understanding and peace among individuals, Pilates' goal echoed these sentiments but in a physical context. He aimed to help individuals attain a strong and balanced body, leading people towards greater self-confidence and self-esteem, enduring health and overall well-being. Just as Jesus empowered the spirit, Pilates empowered the body.

By attempting a synergy between exercise and mindfulness, between toning muscles and mental discipline, Pilates created a fitness regimen that goes beyond mere physical transformation. It echoes the profound tenets of a spiritual journey—self-awareness, deliberate action, inner balance—and leads to a more attuned existence. By understanding the genesis and goal of Pilates, we can better appreciate its holistic approach to wellness and the unlikely parallels to the spiritual teachings of Jesus.

3.4. Bringing It Together: Christ, Pilates, and Ourselves

In summary, the origin and goals of Pilates enable us to see its links to spiritual teaching, particularly that offered by Jesus Christ. Pilates provides us with a way of achieving physical health, enhancing our mental focus, and pursuing a balanced life. Meanwhile, Jesus's teachings parallel such aspirations but on a spiritual level. Both weave together a regimen that strengthens, revitalizes and brings inner peace.

As we embrace the Pilates method and engage with its core principles, we are invited to concurrently embrace the teachings of Jesus, focusing on cultivating greater spiritual strength, compassion, peace and love. In adopting such a lifestyle, we pave the way for a more integrated existence, bringing wellness to our bodies, peace to our minds, and nourishment to our souls.

This journey illustrates how, from a need to rehabilitate physical ailments and a quest for a healthy body, emerged a practice that resonates with one of the world's most profound spiritual teachings. It showcases how resilient the human spirit can be, and how, when the body, mind, and spirit align, one can experience life in its fullest.

In the end, understanding the origins and goals of Pilates serves as a foundation for exploring its extensive application to our holistic well-being—physically, mentally, and spiritually. Today, not just as a robust exercise regimen, Pilates stands at the confluence of our physical health and spiritual journey, offering a path to integrated wellness, inner strength, and profound peace.

Chapter 4. Parallels between Jesus' Teachings and Pilates Principles

The underlying philosophies of Pilates and the teachings of Jesus Christ may seem disparate at first glance. However, when scrutinized closely, striking parallels unearth themselves in the form of principles that both ideologies adhere to - principles rooted deeply in cultivating inner strength, achieving total harmony, and living an enriched and fulfilling life.

4.1. The Essence of Mindfulness

Pilates emphasizes being fully engaged in the moment, with each movement demanding your undivided attention. The exercises' focus is often on one's breathing as it is believed to increase awareness in the body, aiding in synchronization and enhancing effectiveness. This mindfulness is uncannily mirrored in the teachings of Jesus, where He often implores His followers to "Therefore do not worry about tomorrow, for tomorrow will worry about itself. Each day has enough trouble of its own." (Matthew 6:34). A teaching that emphasizes concentrating on the present rather than fretting needlessly about an unpredictable future.

4.2. Unity of Body, Mind, and Spirit

Both Pilates and the teachings of Jesus aim for a harmonious unity of the body, mind, and spirit. Pilates seeks to achieve this through controlled movements, focusing on strength, flexibility, and aerobic conditioning. In essence, it promotes physical well-being to enhance mental clarity. Jesus' teachings, on the other hand, talk about uniting body, mind, and spirit towards the singular purpose of glorifying

God. He states, "Love the Lord your God with all your heart and with all your soul and with all your mind and with all your strength." (Mark 12:30) This verse emphasizes engaging all aspects of oneself in pursuit of divine love and devotion.

4.3. Emphasis on Inner Strength

Just as Pilates stresses the development of core strength, Jesus' teachings emphasize the cultivation of an internal, spiritual strength. Pilates uses a set of controlled movements specifically framed to tighten the body's powerhouse strength—the abdomen, lower back, and pelvic muscles. Likewise, Jesus preached about building inner strength, but His was of a spiritual nature—"But those who hope in the Lord will renew their strength. They will soar on wings like eagles; they will run and not grow weary, they will walk and not be faint." (Isaiah 40:31)

4.4. The Approach of Non-Judgement

Pilates is centered on personal growth and improvement. It requires you to be aware of your body, pushing past limits without judgement. This mirrors Jesus' teachings about casting out judgment and promoting acceptance and understanding. Jesus encourages His followers to look within and rectify their shortcomings before criticizing others - "Do not judge, or you too will be judged."(Matthew 7:1).

4.5. The Practice of Persistence

Both Pilates and Jesus' teachings show significant emphasis on commitment and persistence. Pilates asks for dedication and perseverance, with the understanding that rewards are met after consistent effort. This resonates with Jesus' teachings. He urges His followers to "Ask and it will be given to you; seek and you will find; knock and the door will be opened to you." (Matthew 7:7). The verse emphasizes relentless pursuit—of knowledge, righteousness, and God's mercy.

4.6. Importance of Balance

Balance, both physical and metaphysical, is a cornerstone of Pilates and Jesus' teachings. Pilates helps you improve your balance by reinforcing your core and improving your physical stability. Similarly, the teachings of Jesus Christ advocate the need for balance in life, especially morality-based. He often talked about leading a balanced life in terms of wealth, kindness, and spirituality - "For where your treasure is, there your heart will be also." (Luke 12:34)

As we delve deeper into the understanding of both Pilates and Jesus' teachings, we begin to appreciate their inherent similarities. Both aid in a beautiful exploration of body and spirit that encourages us to become the best versions of ourselves. Indeed, in their unique way, they bring us one step closer to reaching an equilibrium of spiritual strength and physical health.

Chapter 5. The Jesus' Perspective on Physical Wellbeing

In the gospels, we find numerous instances where Jesus pays great attention to the physical wellbeing of individuals around him. His perspective on physical wellness can be seen through his teachings and his actions, emphasizing the importance of taking care of our physical bodies as temples of the Holy Spirit.

5.1. Physical Health as a Sacred Responsibility

According to 1 Corinthians 6:19-20: "Do you not know that your bodies are temples of the Holy Spirit, who is in you, whom you have received from God? You are not your own; you were bought at a price. Therefore honor God with your bodies."

The body's wellness was not peripheral for Jesus but was integrated with his mission. Health is a sacred responsibility, and taking care of our bodies is a way of recognizing and honoring this divine providence. Stewardship involves the fullness of our being – body, mind, and spirit. Physical wellness, essential for fulfilling our life's purpose, firmly roots in our commitment to self-care.

5.2. Jesus, the Healer and His Teachings

Jesus' life offers profound teachings on physical wellbeing. His healing miracles symbolize His compassion and concern for our bodily health.

One of the well-known healing miracles is the story of a paralyzed man in Mark 2:1-12, where faith and the power to heal joined together. Jesus told the man, "Son, your sins are forgiven," and then commanded him to get up, take his bed and walk. While healing his body, Jesus also emphasized the man's spiritual cleansing. This event underscores that Jesus, as a healer, acknowledged the interconnectedness of physical and spiritual wellness.

5.3. The Importance of Rest

Jesus understood the importance of rest and often took time away from the crowds to restore His energy. In Mark 6:31, Jesus tells His disciples, "Come away by yourselves to a secluded place and rest a while." He recognized the importance of self-care, of rejuvenating, replenishing energies and restoring balance to the body, to better serve others.

5.4. Physical Activity and Work as Worship

Jesus also emphasized the role of physical work as part of spiritual practice. As a carpenter, He set an example that physical work our bodies perform can also be a form of worship. This approach can lend a new perspective to our Pilates regimen, which involves using the body's strength, flexibility, and endurance. Positioning it as an act of devotion aligns with Jesus' teachings and can bring a deeper sense of meaning to the practice.

5.5. Influence of Diet on Physical Wellbeing

The Bible also presents examples of Jesus acknowledging the role of diet in maintaining physical wellbeing. The "Life Bread" narrative

(John 6:35) implies that, while it is essential that we rely on God for our spiritual nourishment, we also must take care of our physical bodies by maintaining a balanced and healthy diet.

In conclusion, Jesus's perspective on physical wellbeing isn't a standalone concept. It interlinks the body's wellness with a wholesome approach that caters to spiritual, emotional, and mental health. He encourages us to embrace physical health not merely as an aesthetic endeavor but as an active part of the overall wellbeing, the improvement of which can enhance spiritual connectivity. As we engage in Pilates, we're not just training our bodies, but also deepening our spiritual relationships, connecting with the teachings of Jesus, and embodying His perspective on physical wellness. By embracing this holistic strategy, we can enrich our lives with a fulfilling interaction between faith, mind, and body – a lifestyle Jesus himself demonstrated.

Chapter 6. Spiritual Lessons from Pilates Postures

Pilates, as a physical discipline aimed at improving balance, strength, and flexibility, engages both the body and mind. Its techniques bear uncanny resemblances to timeless spiritual truths propagated by Jesus. Drawing parallels, we dive into the world of spiritual enlightenment through Pilates postures and their symbolic meanings.

6.1. The Hundred Posture: Lessons in Tenacity and Perseverance

Roman Pilates designed the Hundred posture to build strength and endurance. It represents the human struggle against adversities. Similarly, Jesus emphasized perseverance in His teachings. He held that life wasn't free from tribulations (John 16:33), rather, one must persevere through trials to find joy and peace.

In the Hundred posture, you maintain a controlled breathing pattern, similar to meditative practices. Results don't come instantly; they demand diligence and consistency. Allowing the struggles to shape rather than break you is the path to spiritual maturity, embodied by Jesus's crucifixion and resurrection.

6.2. Bridge Posture: A Lesson in Connection and Unity

The Bridge posture, which elevates the core off the floor, symbolizes the bridge connecting our physical selves to our spiritual essence. It represents an attempt to seek unity within the self and the world around. In the same vein, Jesus taught about unity and connection. In

John 17:21, He prayed his disciples would be one, just like He and his Father were one.

Performing this posture prompts introspection, encouraging us to be conduits of goodness and light, mirroring Jesus's call to be reflections of God's love. This posture also activates the heart chakra, relating closely to the virtue of love, a cardinal theme in Jesus's teachings.

6.3. Teaser Posture: Balance and Equilibrium

The Teaser posture embodies equilibrium, encouraging both physical and mental balance. This aligns with the teachings of Jesus, who fostered harmony and balance in His life. In the Gospel of Mark (12:31), Jesus calls us to love our neighbors as we love ourselves, underscoring the importance of balance between self-care and care for others.

This posture is hard to hold, implying that maintaining balance in life often requires effort. We must constantly work to balance personal growth with service to others, worldly responsibilities with spiritual ones.

6.4. Saw Posture: Removing Spiritual Blindness

The Saw posture stretches your body forcing your gaze past your extended hand, symbolizing the removal of spiritual blindness. It aligns with the story in John 9 where Jesus heals a man born blind, allowing him to see both physically and spiritually.

Pilates calls us to be internally attentive and intentional about our movements as Jesus's teachings urge us to be aware of our spiritual sight. This pose implores us to cut away false notions and prejudices, enabling a clearer perception of truth.

6.5. Child's Pose: Lessons in Surrender and Humility

Child's Pose signifies surrendering to a higher power and humbling ourselves, a lesson Jesus emphasized in Matthew 18:4 – "Whoever humbles himself like this child is the greatest in the Kingdom of Heaven."

Engaging in this restorative pose, we learn the value of stillness, quietness, and acceptance. We find relief through surrender, recalling Jesus's invitation (Matthew 11:28-30) to those weary and burdened to find rest in Him.

Incorporating these spiritual teachings within our physical exercises could enhance our mental resilience while strengthening our faith. The parallels between Pilates and Jesus's teachings are a testament to the universal wisdom that promotes internal and external harmony. As we navigate through life, let's coil and stretch, stand tall and lean low, exploring the depths of our spiritual potential with hope, faith, and unyielding vigour.

Chapter 7. Breathwork: Embracing the Holy Spirit through Pilates

The teachings of Jesus inspire the heart and soothe the soul, while Pilates strengthens the body and invigorates the mind. A convergence of these two influences can bring about inner harmony, aligning the breath with spirit. This chapter explores the importance of breathwork in Pilates and its spiritual parallelism in the teachings of Jesus, drawing upon the perspective of embracing the Holy Spirit.

7.1. A Primer to Breathwork in Pilates

We need to start this journey, fundamentally, with an understanding of breathwork in Pilates. It's a cornerstone of the practice, used to connect with one's body, to fuel the movements, and to focus the mind. Pilates breathwork is typically categorized into lateral or thoracic breathing, which differs from the everyday breathing we're accustomed to. This method involves deeply inhaling through the nose, filling the sides and back of the ribcage, and exhaling fully through pursed lips, gently contracting the abdominal muscles.

In this process, breath becomes more than just a life-sustaining function—it morphs into a powerful tool that orchestrates the rhythm and delivery of each Pilates movement. By learning to harness the power of your breath in this manner, you are taking the initial step in your unique journey towards a harmonious integration of body, mind, and spirit.

7.2. The Holy Spirit in Christian Teachings

Now that we have comprehended the essence of breathwork in Pilates, let's explore its spiritual counterpart. In Christian belief, breath has significant spiritual connotations. The Hebrew word 'ruach,' used in the Bible, often interchanges between 'wind,' 'breath,' and 'spirit.' The word's different interpretations signify the Holy Spirit, the divine life force, representing God's active presence in the world.

In the New Testament, Jesus speaks of the Holy Spirit in parallels to the wind, highlighting its unseen yet powerful presence, much like the breath in our bodies. In John 3:8, Jesus said, "The wind blows wherever it pleases. You hear its sound, but you cannot tell where it comes from or where it is going. So it is with everyone born of the Spirit." This metaphorical assessment endorses the significance of breath as a representation of the Holy Spirit that flows within us.

7.3. Unifying the Breath and the Spirit

The parallels between breathwork in Pilates and the Holy Spirit's significance in Christian teachings offer a beautiful integration of the body and spirit. By consciously engaging with our breath during Pilates, we can create a kindred connection to the Holy Spirit, embracing its presence within us.

As we inhale, filling our ribcage expansively and revitalizing each cell, we invite the Holy Spirit to fill us with love, peace, and resilience. As we exhale, contracting our abdomen and expelling every bit of air, we release our doubts, fears, and stresses, surrendering them to God. This active interaction exhilaratingly transforms our Pilates practice into a lived experience of prayer and meditation.

7.4. Breathwork Exercises for Embracing the Holy Spirit

Breathwork isn't merely about inhaling and exhaling; it's an essential element of exercising control over your body. Below are some exercises that synergize Pilates and the spiritual teachings of Jesus, fostering a deeper connection with the Holy Spirit as part of your fitness regime.

1. Hundred Breathing: This breathing technique is named after the Pilates Hundred exercise, which is composed of 100 breath cycles. Start by inhaling for five counts while performing precise arm movements, then exhale for five counts. As you execute this exercise, consider each breath as an invitation for the Holy Spirit to fill you. Each distinctive exhale can serve as a prayer, or a release of the things that hold you back, enabling spiritual growth and bodily strength in synchrony.

2. Lateral Breathing: Lateral or thoracic breathing not only refines your Pilates technique but also amplifies mindfulness. As you breathe in deeply, filling your sides and back of your ribcage, visualize the Holy Spirit filling you with divine energy. With each exhalation, envision the release of all tension, worries, and negativity.

3. Box Breathing: Also known as square breathing, this technique calms the nervous system and enhances focus. Begin with inhaling, holding your breath, exhaling, and pausing your breath again, all to the count of five. As you engage in this pattern, attune your attention to the guiding presence of the Holy Spirit. Use each pause to reflect on your blessings, embedding a sense of gratitude within your core.

7.5. Reflective Practice: Anchoring Yourself in the Breath

This enriching amalgamation of breathwork in Pilates and embracing the Holy Spirit is akin to a moving meditation, a reflective practice invigorating both body and spirit. Resting in the rhythm of your breath, surrendering to the flowing wind of the Spirit, and feeling the ebb and flow of divine energy within your being, you anchor yourself in the present moment.

Embracing the Holy Spirit through Pilates thus becomes an empowering experience, a unique approach to holistic wellness that echoes resonantly within your being long after the exercise session has concluded.

"The Spirit of God has made me; the breath of the Almighty gives me life." (Job 33:4). These holy words enshrine an essential truth that can elevate our perspective of the practice of Pilates. As we embrace this convergence of breathwork and spiritual consciousness, we discover an elevated sense of well-being, holistic rejuvenation, and a renewed connection with our Divine essence. This practice not only keeps our bodies physically fit but also enriches our spiritual life, making us healthier, happier, and more in tune with the divine existence that breathes within us.

Chapter 8. The Power of Mindfulness: Reflections from Pilates and The Bible

Mindfulness is a term often associated with meditation and yoga. It is a practice that teaches us to live in the present moment, aware of our thoughts, feelings, and actions but not consumed by them. It is an approach that can greatly enrich our spiritual life, as well as our physical well-being. A concept that finds resonance both in the physicality of Pilates and the teachings from The Bible.

8.1. The Concept of Mindfulness in Pilates

Joseph Pilates, the creator of Pilates, premised the practice on the idea of complete coordination of the body, mind, and spirit. Mindfulness comes into play as the sense of full presence and conscious effort in each movement. Performing Pilates exercises requires intense concentration, engaging your mind fully, aligning it with the rhythm of your breath and the precision of your movements. The idea is not just to move but to 'experience the movement,' fostering a profound connection between the physical and mental self.

Pilates teaches the difference between just 'doing' actions, and 'being' in the actions. The difference lies in awareness, and this awareness fosters presence. Josef Pilates once said, "It is the mind itself that builds the body." Each movement in Pilates, when done mindfully, strengthens the neuromuscular pathways, aiding not just the physical strength, but also enhancing mental clarity and control.

8.2. Mindfulness Within The Bible's Teachings

While the term 'mindfulness' is not explicitly used in The Bible, the ideals appear throughout its teachings. Scriptures repeatedly urge us to focus, to be alert, to meditate on God's word, to be conscious of our actions and thoughts.

In Matthew 6:34, Jesus said, "Therefore do not worry about tomorrow, for tomorrow will worry about itself. Each day has enough trouble of its own." Jesus understood the futile anxiety that entraps us when we ponder the past or future. He urged us to be present, to trust God's provision, indicating the essence of mindfulness.

Likewise, passages such as Psalm 46:10, "Be still, and know that I am God," direct us to be mindful, to quiet our thoughts, and realize the omnipresence of God. It is a call to settle into the quiet awareness of divine presence.

The Bible encourages us to remain focused, attentive, and committed in prayer: "Rejoice always, pray without ceasing, give thanks in all circumstances" (1 Thessalonians 5:16-18). This scriptural guidance is akin to mindfulness meditation, where we train our focus and awareness.

8.3. Mindfulness: The Confluence Of Physical And Spiritual Wellness

Mindfulness in Pilates and teachings from The Bible may seem disparate at the surface, but upon closer look, we witness a unifying thread. Both practices promote mindfulness to foster a rich connection with the body and spirit, allowing us to thrive fully in the present moment.

The constant emphasis on mindfulness in Pilates builds muscular strength and flexibility while also training the mind to be alert, clear, and focused. Bridging the gap between physical exertion and mindful meditation, Pilates perfectly marries the benefits of both worlds, leading to comprehensive wellness.

In conjunction, The Bible guides us to mindfulness in our spiritual life. It encourages us to be present, to meditate on God's word, to align our thoughts and actions with His teachings. This mindfulness enables us to cultivate deeper relations with God, fostering spiritual growth and mental peace.

8.4. How To Incorporate Mindfulness In Our Daily Lives

Although the context of mindfulness differs in The Bible and Pilates, the essence remains the same, and this essence can be integrated into daily life. Here's a practical approach to get started:

1. Be Present: While performing a task, focus completely on it. For example, feel the sensation of brushing your teeth, the water, the paste, the motion. It may sound trivial, but it's a simple exercise in mindfulness.

2. Deep Breathing: Whenever you feel overwhelmed, take a moment to breathe deeply. With each exhale, imagine stress leaving your body and mind. This helps center your thoughts.

3. Body Scan: At any point in the day, close your eyes and scan your body mentally. Start from your toes and go up to your head. Feel each part of your body, notice any tension, discomfort, or relaxation.

4. Meditate on Scripture: Select a passage from The Bible, read it slowly, meditate on every word, and try to understand its essence. How does it apply to your life today? Reflect on that.

5. Practice Gratitude: Practicing gratitude is an act of mindfulness. Before sleeping, write down three things you're grateful for. This reflection helps retain a positive mindset.

8.5. Concluding Thoughts

Embracing mindfulness in our daily lives, just as Pilates and The Bible encourage, opens up a pathway of harmony both in our physical bodies and spiritual selves. It fosters a deep sense of awareness that enables us not just to live, but to live fully, appreciating the present moment, fostering gratitude, and navigating stress with grace and strength. As we learn to strengthen our mindfulness muscles with the wisdom drawn from Pilates and The Bible, we fashion an enriching life, tailored to bolster our physical, mental, and spiritual wellness.

Through this journey, we truly understand the profundity of the interconnectedness of body, mind, and spirit, leading us to realize that the key to holistic wellness lies within us, within this very moment; we merely need to be aware and mindful of it.

Chapter 9. Building Core Strength: Physical and Spiritual

Our journey through enhancing fitness and faith begins with two essential cornerstones: physical and spiritual core strength. As the epicenter of human balance and foundation, the physical core is critical to implementing Pilates' techniques effectively. Likewise, the spiritual core–our inner faith–serves as the essence of our relationship with the divine, predominantly embedding the teachings of Jesus Christ. Together, this blend of physical prowess and spiritual enlightenment can significantly reimagine our approach to holistic wellness.

9.1. Understanding Physical Core Strength

The human body's core consists of several muscles spanning the abdomen, lower back, and hips. These muscle groups play an essential role in maintaining balance, promoting good posture, ensuring efficient movement and guarding against injuries. In Pilates, the core—often referred to as the 'powerhouse'—is where all movements initiates and radiate outward. Consequently, an efficient core workout can not only provide an aesthetically pleasing physique but also lead to a sense of overall physical well-being.

To build our physical core strength, let's start with some fundamental Pilates exercises.

1. **The Hundred:** Distinguished as a significant warming-up exercise, it engages your abdominal muscles, helping maintain a controlled breathing rhythm.

2. **Knee Folds:** Engage your lower abdominal muscles with this simple but effective move, guiding your body to achieve balance and control in motion.

3. **Plank:** This comprehensive exercise engages every part of your core, promoting better posture and overall physical strength.

Remember, consistency is vital when it comes to physical workouts, and the focus should always be on practicing effectively rather than measuring the number of repetitions or duration. Over time, the improved core strength wouldn't just be evident in your toned physique but would also mirror in your daily activities—from the way you walk to your increased stamina.

9.2. The Significance of Spiritual Core Strength

Parallel to fortifying our physical core lies the task of nurturing our spiritual core. In the context of our journey, the spiritual core refers to our relationship with God—as shaped by the teachings of Jesus, nurtured by faith, prayer, virtue and a heart full of love.

A strong spiritual core provides an unwavering foundation in times of trials, nourishing hope and resilience. It embellishes our life with virtues such as forgiveness, charity, and humility–all of them constituting Christ's teachings. There are myriad ways to strengthen our spiritual core:

1. **Daily Prayer:** Make prayer a daily habit. Through constant communication with the divine, you are likely to experience the strengthening of your faith, deepening your connection with God.

2. **Studying Scriptures:** The Bible is a treasure trove of wisdom. Regular reading and meditating on its verses can anchor our lives, providing us with spiritual sustenance and fortifying our spiritual core.

3. **Love and Service:** Implementing Christ's teaching of 'loving your neighbor as yourself' into action reinforces our spiritual core, making it more strong and resilient.

4. **Community Involvement:** Actively participating in community events or church-based activities often facilitates spiritual growth and fortifies our spiritual core.

9.3. Synthesizing Physical and Spiritual Strength

While seemingly disparate, working on our physical and spiritual cores can have a synergistic effect, enhancing the development of each other. As one becomes increasingly aware of their physical strength and ability, it can inspire a sense of gratitude towards the divine – resulting in a motivated effort to nourish their spiritual core.

Similarly, a well-nurtured spiritual core can inject perseverance and discipline in maintaining and achieving physical fitness goals. The patience, dedication, and resilience instilled by spiritual practices transcend in maintaining consistency in physical exercises.

Connecting this synthesis back to our broader scope of holistic wellness, we can observe that a balanced development of our physical and spiritual cores results in a thoughtful blend of physical well-being and spiritual rejuvenation—leading us closer to the comprehensive wellness we seek.

There's a distinct kind of empowerment that comes from the fusion of physical and spiritual core strengthening—a combination of the robustness of the body and resilience of the spirit. This empowerment is a beacon that guides us through life's struggles, encouraging us to emerge stronger and wiser. Here's to the building of that core strength, the foundation of our journey towards holistic wellness. Through this journey, we aim to mirror the teachings of Jesus Christ, grounding us in faith, and Pilates, grounding us in strength.

As you continue to explore and experience this harmonious relationship, remember to be patient. Progress is often gradual and requires consistent effort. This journey towards a stronger core–both physical and spiritual–is less of a destination but more of a path of continuous growth, self-discovery, and enlightenment. So, embark on this journey with a heart full of hope, a mind full of curiosity, and a spirit full of determination.

Chapter 10. Healing and Transformation: Pilates and Faith

The amalgamation of Pilates and faith is not as farfetched as it may initially seem. Both disciplines encourage the practitioner to delve deep within themselves, strengthening their understanding and fortitude while discovering new spiritual realities. This pervasive, life-reshaping experience is enlightened by Jesus' teachings, which are filled with wisdom and goodwill.

10.1. The Intersecting Pathways

The first step towards the practice of healing and transformation is to understand the intersecting pathways of Pilates and faith. While Pilates primarily comments on physical fitness, its underlying goal is to refine and develop the mind, paralleling faith's purpose.

Pilates, developed by Joseph Pilates in the early 20th century, focuses on controlled movements, balance, and flexibility primarily for the core muscles – which include the abdomen, lower back, and hips. The essence of Pilates lies in the conscious control of all muscular movements. The system emphasises precision, concentration, and breathing, with a strong mind and body connection. Every movement is believed to originate from the core and then radiate outwards.

Faith, particularly when discussing Jesus' teachings, is equally transformative, emphasizing the strengthening of spiritual connections and the renewal of the inner self. Jesus' teachings involve virtues such as love, forgiveness, and faith itself, guiding us towards a path of self-understanding and spiritual enlightenment.

10.2. The Embodiment of Healing

The physical benefits of Pilates are well-documented and widely recognized: a strengthened core, improved flexibility, better posture, and enhanced bodily control. However, what often gets overlooked is the potential for healing that Pilates holds - from alleviating chronic pain to assisting with injury recovery. This art form enforces a state of mindfulness that facilitates body awareness and fosters physical healing.

Faith plays a similar role but on the spiritual level. The teachings of Jesus imbue us with a sense of hope, perseverance, love, and camaraderie. We are instructed to believe without seeing—an act of faith that often brings miraculous healing to challenging life situations.

10.3. Sacred Breathing

In Pilates, breathing is more than a process of oxygen exchange. It is an essential method that dictates the rhythm and intensity of every movement, helping to center focus and attention while performing the exercises. Conscious breathing during workout sessions allows for better muscular control and coordination, thus enabling the practitioner to achieve a more efficient and beneficial workout.

Similarly, in the spiritual context, the breath is considered sacred and life-giving. In Genesis 2:7, the Bible records: "Then the Lord God formed a man from the dust of the ground and breathed into his nostrils the breath of life, and the man became a living being." Breathing is a sign of the divine spirit within us - a constant reminder of God's pervasive presence.

10.4. The Act of Surrender

Surrender forms another unique intersection between Pilates and faith. In Pilates, surrendering refers to letting go of physical tension and allowing the body to align naturally to execute movements effectively. Outwardly, it may seem simple, but this act requires significant mental effort and self-awareness.

In faith, surrendering extends beyond the physical realm to the spiritual realm. It involves submitting to God's will and acknowledging His sovereign power and wisdom. The act of relinquishing control to God uplifts the spirit and can aid in navigating through trials and tribulations.

10.5. Mindfulness and Meditation

Finally, the aspect of mindfulness and meditation encompasses both Pilates and faith. Pilates cultivates mindfulness by centering a person's attention on their movements, breathing, and bodily sensations. The movements are performed with conscious attention and intention, promoting an enhanced sense of body awareness and self-control.

In the spiritual realm, meditation plays a crucial role. Jesus frequently retreated to private places to pray and meditate, a practice amplified in Christianity. Meditating on God's word, immersing in prayer, and cultivating mindfulness of His presence strengthens believers' connection with the divine.

10.6. Conclusion: The Complete Transformation

Bringing together the robust physical exercise of Pilates with the spiritual insights endowed by faith provides a comprehensive and balanced approach to health and wellness. This harmonious blending facilitates a complete transformation - strengthening the body, enhancing mental capacity, and enriching the spirit.-

Chapter 11. Cultivating a Pilates-inspired Spiritual Routine

The fusion of physical well-being with spiritual enlightenment forms the philosophy at the core of this transformative routine. Here, we'll unfold how you can integrate the core strengthening principles of Pilates with the spiritual profundity of Jesus' teachings to develop a comprehensive regimen for holistic wellness.

11.1. Understanding the Foundations: Pilates and Spirituality

To cultivate a Pilates-inspired spiritual routine, one must first appreciate the respective roles of Pilates and spirituality in our lives. Pilates is a physical fitness system developed in the early 20th century by Joseph Pilates. This system centers around core strength and flexibility, boasting a multitude of benefits such as improved posture, muscle tone, balance, and joint health.

Simultaneously, spiritual life, especially in the context of Jesus' life and teachings, provides a profound sense of purpose and inner peace. His lessons of love, forgiveness, and perseverance offer a moral and ethical compass to navigate through life's complexities.

Bringing Pilates and spirituality together allows for a comprehensive wellness strategy that can strengthen the body while centering the mind and spirit.

11.2. Commencing the Routine: Beginning with Prayer

The most effective way to initiate your Pilates-inspired spiritual routine is through prayer. Begin by expressing gratitude, seeking guidance, or simply communicating with God. This process fosters mindfulness which tunes your awareness into the present moment, an aspect critical to practicing Pilates.

Use the following prayer as a starting point or craft your own motivational invocation:

```
Dear God,
Guide me as I embark on this journey of growth and
change,
Please let each movement cleanse my body and open my
heart to your sacred teachings.
Amen.
```

11.3. Integration into Practice: Pilates and Scripture

One unique aspect of this routine is to pair physical exercises with relevant scriptural reflections. When engaging in Pilates, imagine each exercise serving as a metaphorical embodiment of a certain aspect of the teachings of Jesus. As you strengthen your core, consider that you're also strengthening your spiritual core.

Begin with a set of basic Pilates exercises:

- The Pilates Hundred

- Roll Up

- Single Leg Circles

- Rolling Like a Ball

- Single Leg Stretch

- Double Leg Stretch

- Criss-Cross

Now, couple each exercise with a relevant scripture from the Bible. For example, while performing the 'Roll Up', you may pair it with Philippians 4:13 "I can do all things through Christ who strengthens me". Allow this scripture to be your mantra. Repeat it in your mind as you perform the exercise. The idea is to associate the physical strength and resilience you build with the exercise with the moral and spiritual strength symbolized by the scripture.

This integration enables a deeper connection with your spiritual component.

11.4. Creating Spiritual Rhythms: Breathwork in Pilates

Breathwork plays a significant role in Pilates, as coordinated breathing is used to enhance movements. Each exercise emphasizes deep, controlled breathing, and the exhale typically coordinates with the most strenuous part of the exercise.

You can use breathe as a bridge between physical exercises and spirituality. As you engage in the Pilates Hundred, feel your entire being fill with life-giving oxygen as you inhale, then exhale, releasing any physical and emotional tensions. Remember Genesis 2:7, where God breathes life into man. Through our breathing, we are intrinsically linked with our Creator.

11.5. Nurturing Silence: Rest and Reflection

At the end of your routine, set aside time for rest and reflection, akin to the 'still' phases in Pilates. This time provides a space for relaxation and introspection, where you can deepen spiritual connections and internalize the wisdom from the chosen scriptures.

Meditate on how the physical aspects of the routine paralleled the spiritual lessons. Simple questions to contemplate could be: how has this exercise helped strengthen my faith? What changes have I noticed in my body, thoughts, or emotions?

11.6. Adapting the Routine

This Pilates-inspired spiritual routine is not a rigid regimen but a flexible and adaptable framework. Every individual is unique, so you can adjust this routine to better fit your personal spiritual journey and fitness level. As you progress, try incorporating more advanced Pilates exercises and aligning them with different scriptures that speak to you.

By consciously uniting the physical and spiritual components in this pilgrimage of well-being, you'll be embracing a holistic approach to wellness that strengthens your body, kindles your mind, and enlivens your spirit. Above all remember, wellness is a personal journey. Yours, then, is to find a spiritual routine that not only challenges you but also nurtures you- physically, mentally, and spiritually. Cultivating a Pilates-inspired spiritual routine is about harmoniously unifying the essence of physical strength and spiritual awareness to foster a fulfilled and vibrant life.